Generosity: The Perfect Drug

10 Incredible Benefits of Giving

By Douglas M. Clark

This book is dedicated to my partners in the effort to live a generous life:

Sheila
Greg
Ted
David
Lyle
Katie

Contents

PREFACE

I believe that all of us have an innate desire to be generous. For some, that desire is fully awake. For some, it lies dormant. For others, it occasionally raises it's head and is acted on, for several reasons, drops below the surface again. I, too, have a desire to be generous – to live a passionately generous life.

Believe me, it isn't always easy. There are challenges, obstacles blocking our way to being generous. Living a generous life is not 'convenient.'

Every morning an alarm goes off on my phone with the following notification:

G3=L!

It looks like some kind of algebraic formula. Here is what the equation means.

The letter G stands for 'Give.'

The number '3' symbolizes the three resources that I have:

> Time,
> Talent (abilities), and
> Treasure (money).
> '=' stands for equals (no brainer)
> The letter L stands for 'Live.'

Put in a sentence, it would read:

"When I give of my time, talent, and treasure, I come alive!"

I have learned that life is more than getting, accumulating, and owning.

Do you remember how you felt the last time you gave something to someone or did something for someone? Wasn't that a great feeling? Wouldn't you like to feel that way every day?

You can!

In this book, we will look at the incredible benefits of generosity. I hope that as you read it, you will be moved to live a passionately generous life. A generous life is the most exciting way to live, for it is in giving that we truly come alive.

I want to say a special thanks to my Board Members - passionately generous life. Sheila, Katie, David, Ted, Greg, Lyle, who were my proofreaders and who daily strive to live a generous life. You are an inspiration to me.

Generosity is the Perfect Drug!

Doug

4

INTRODUCTION

Drugs

Aren't they wonderful?

If you watch television, even for just a little while, you will see that there seems to be a drug for every issue under the sun. Many of which I have never even heard of.

Whatever the issue, there is a drug to help. If you have a headache, are giving birth, are ill, can't breathe, have a chemical imbalance – no matter what, there seems to be a drug that can help.

Lucky us!

That is until you hear the voice at the end of the commercial that has just extolled the virtues of the latest and greatest drug:

"Side effects may include rashes, bleeding, high blood pressure, risk of clots, nervousness, paranoia, headaches, loss of sight, loss of hearing, incontinence, depression, suicidal thoughts, inability to swallow, and more!"

By the end of the disclaimer, you ask yourself, "Is the drug worse than the disease?"

If only there were a perfect drug that didn't have these incredible side effects.

I have good news for you, there is!

Yes, you read correctly. There is a Perfect Drug that has no side effects. A drug that cures many of the maladies that you and I suffer from daily.

Yes, I know, I could hardly believe it myself.

What is that drug? Well, you might laugh when I tell you. And legally, I must add this disclaimer: the FDA has not cleared it as a product they can support (or regulate).

That drug is "Generosity!"

Stick with me, friend. Let me explain how I concluded that Generosity is the Perfect Drug.

My first inclination about generosity was from the belief that you might relate with. I gave and thought everyone should give because basically, it was a good thing to do. Plain and simple! You know, the Golden Rule:

"Do (give) unto others as you would have them do (give) unto you!"

Or the other belief that spurred me to be generous, if I was to be completely honest, was a bit more self-serving. Maybe if you were to be really honest you could relate with me and admit that you always, often or sometimes give for the following reason:

"Give, and it shall be given back to you!"

This reason for giving is good. In fact, it is excellent. But, as I looked further into generosity, I was pleasantly surprised to find there were HUGE benefits to giving.

There are more significant reasons to give than just because it is a good thing to do.

There are Benefits that I can experience and benefits that others can experience.

Benefits so high that an individual's physical, mental, emotional, and spiritual wellbeing improved when they gave.

That is when I began calling Generosity 'The Perfect Drug!'.

There are no harmful side effects! No 'downside' to living generously. Yep, you read correctly!

There is no risk of increased rashes, bleeding, high blood pressure, clots, nervousness, paranoia, headaches, loss of sight, loss of hearing, incontinence, depression, suicidal thoughts, inability to swallow....yada yada.

There are only positive side effects. Ten of which I present in the following chapters: 5 benefits to others and 5 benefits to you!

So, if you are interested in that kind of drug read on!

One of my hopes is that by the time you are finished reading this book, your giving meter will have been nudged up even if just a smidgen.

However, the truth be told, my real desire is to start a movement, a Generosity Cartel if you will, with syndicates everywhere. A Cartel full of passionate believers who extol its virtues, demonstrate its impact, distribute it everywhere, and get everyone hooked on it. Yep, in essence, you read correctly. It boils down to this: I am a drug dealer, and I invite you to join me!

"Life's most persistent and urgent question is,
what are you doing for others?"

Dr. Martin Luther King Jr

Chapter 1

Charcoal Please!

I have a friend (we will call him Carlos) who lives in a developing country – an impoverished developing country, and he came from the poorest of the poor. Growing up in the slums of the capital city, each day was a struggle to find enough money to purchase food to stay alive.

He has a family of his own now and feels the daily weight of providing for them. Finding ways to do so is not easy. He can't just walk to the corner fast food joint and get a minimum wage job – there is no fast food joint. And there is no minimum wage.

There is, however, a central market.

Every day people bring their wares and their produce to sell. One of the things they sell are tortillas. Ladies will sit over a charcoal fire for hours, making tortillas then take them to market to sell. However, charcoal is hard to locate and even harder to transport since most don't have a vehicle.

My friend came up with an idea. He knew where to get charcoal. He would set up an account with the charcoal vendor, transport the charcoal to the market, and sell it to the tortilla makers so that they could make tortillas. In so doing, he could make money to buy food for his own family.

Great idea!

The problem: Just like everyone else, he had no way to transport the charcoal from the vendor to the market. He didn't let that deter him. He began saving every penny he could until he had enough to purchase a three-wheeled motorcycle that had a cargo box on the back of it.

When I became aware of his project, he had been at it a while. He hadn't even raised a fraction of the money necessary to purchase the moto-cargo vehicle.

I felt inclined to assist. I reached out to Carlos and committed to help him.

Soon after, my entrepreneurial friend had a basic yet beautiful vehicle that he could use to transport the charcoal. This simple act, on my part, encouraged him, filled him with optimism, and met his need for a vehicle. He became the 'Charcoal Supplier' in his community.

So, what's the first benefit that is realized by giving?

Let's start with the basic, no brainer.The first benefit of Giving is:

A need is met!

"Duh," you might say, "it doesn't take a rocket scientist to figure that out!"

While this is the obvious result of giving, we don't want to overlook the fact that it is indeed a benefit to giving.

Because there is always the: 'What if!?!'

Have you ever thought of that?

What would happen if, when given the opportunity, you did not give?

What happens to that need?

Yes, someone else may give, but what if they don't? Or what if they do? But it takes resources, time, and abilities away from the need they had planned to give to?

Think of the ripple effect.

Someone somewhere is going to have a need that doesn't get met – or someone is going to have to 'give double' to cover for the person who didn't give.

Now let's go back to what happens when we do give. What is the significant immediate effect on people's lives?

Their need is met.

There are few things as wondrous, as comforting, as life-giving than when a need is met.

Have you ever had a need met?

Meaning, have you ever had something in your life that needed to get done, and you could not do it yourself?

For example:

- Have you ever needed to pay the rent, and you just didn't have the money?

- Have you ever needed to buy groceries, and you just didn't have the money for food?

- Have you ever needed to lift something on to a shelf, but it was too heavy for just one person?

- Have you ever needed to buy clothes for your children and not had the money to purchase them?

- Have you ever been in a conundrum, and you needed someone's time so that you could bounce an idea off them?

You know what that felt like. You felt helpless, embarrassed, frustrated, stymied.

It seemed like you couldn't see past that need. You could not accomplish anything else because this need was staring at you in the face consuming all your energy.

Have you ever had someone else reach out and meet that need?

Do you remember what it felt like?

That need, which had become such a weight on your shoulders, was suddenly gone.

And the result of that one action of your need being met was almost magical. The clouds lifted, you could see past today, you began to think optimistically about the future.

Just think, that is what you can do for someone else!

By simply opening your heart – calendar, energy, resources – you can make someone's day.

You can meet a need.

That is benefit #1.

Hang on, there's more, and it gets even better!

Just give!

"What we have done for ourselves alone dies with us; what we have done for others and the world remains and is immortal."

Albert Pike

Chapter 2

Change the Future!

A significant benefit of giving is you can Change the Future!

"Clark, you just took a big jump from the Basic benefit of 'A need being met!' to 'Change the future!' Maybe we should take a breath and sit down and make sure that you are okay!"

Okay, okay, I know it is a big jump, but stay with me; I think I can back this up.

As we discussed in the previous chapter, while the primary effect of giving may 'simply' be that the person is encouraged. Or the underlying effect of giving 'simply' met the

23

basic need for transport by an up and coming charcoal supplier.

What if our giving did more than just 'simply' give a renewed optimism for that day?

What if our giving was more than 'simply' putting wind beneath the wings of an aspiring entrepreneur?

What is the potential long-term effect of your giving to someone's life?

'Simply'' could actually be pretty huge.

Because you gave, charcoal was bought and sold, and a father could purchase food for his family, and as a result, they didn't starve to death. How about that for a 'simple' result?

What if your gift encouraged a person who was so distraught that they were about to call it quits? Because you gave, he did not commit suicide. 'Simply' is now huge.

What if your gift kept the electricity on at someone's house just long enough so that when the severe winter storm hit, they didn't freeze to death? Because you gave, a family did not freeze to death, and the children at the house did not die. Instead, they grew up!

In case that isn't enough, let's continue imagining.

The young girl that lived in that house grew up and went to college. In college, she studied alternative power systems. She then invented an emergency system that would continue to heat a home for 24 hours if the power goes off due to a severe storm.

What is the potential impact on society?

Because you gave, that alternative power system was invented. As a result, the rate of people who freeze to death due to lack of power each year drops to zero.

At this point, you may be saying, 'Whoa Clark, now you are going to far. I was willing to hang with you through the other 'potential impacts', but that is a pretty out of this world hypothetical!"

Yes, you are right, I am letting my imagination carry me away. Most of our giving won't have this impact....or will it?

Stick with me. Watch this...

In 1947 Reverend Robert Pierce met Tena Hoelkedoer, a teacher, while on a trip to China. She introduced him to a battered and abandoned child named White Jade. Unable to care for the child herself, she asked, "What are you going to do about her?" Rev. Pierce gave the woman his last five dollars and agreed to send the same amount each month to help the woman care for the girl.

This encounter was a turning point for Robert. He began building an organization dedicated to helping the world's children. The first child sponsorship program began three years later in response to the needs of hundreds of thousands of orphans at the end of the Korean War.

Over the next several decades, their reach expanded throughout Asia, Latin America, Africa, the Middle East, and Eastern Europe.

In the 1970s, they embraced a broader community development model and established an emergency relief division. They also began attempting to address the causes of poverty by focusing on community needs such as water, sanitation, education, health, leadership training, and income generation.

With the start of the 21st century, they began strengthening their advocacy efforts, particularly on issues related to child survival. They became more active in working with governments, businesses, and other organizations in addressing issues such as child labor, children in armed conflict, and the sexual exploitation of women and children.

Today that organization, which you and I know as World Vision, together with its microfinance subsidiary - is one of the world's leading humanitarian organizations. Over 40,000 staff members implement programs of community development, emergency relief, and promotion of justice in nearly 100 countries.

Okay, let's not lose sight of the trees because of the forest. While we do not know what happened to White Jade, we do know what has happened to others.

Meet George Ndung'u Kamua.

As a young boy in Trans Nzoia, Kenya, George's family lived in complete poverty. His parents struggled to make enough money to provide food and other basic needs. When he was eight years old, someone started sponsoring him. Because of that sponsorship, he received access to education and healthcare.

He graduated at the top of his class and went on to post-graduate studies, ultimately

28

ending up at Harvard. He has become a published author and an expert in Social Protection (cash transfers in emergencies), HIV and AIDS, social accountability, governance, and education.

Listen to what he has to say about someone giving. "I will forever be grateful for the opportunities I have had and recognize how different my life would have been."

It all started with $5.00!

Here is another story about how giving can affect destiny.

When I was young, I lived in Paraguay. In that country, when you stop at a stoplight, you are swarmed by little boys wanting a handout thinly veiled in the form of a service of washing your windshield.

It actually was quite frustrating. Most of the time, the cleaning utensils these boys used were so dirty that they often left more debris and smears of crud when they were done than what was there originally.

As a result, often you would pay them so that they wouldn't wash your windshield.

Anyway, one day, my dad pulled up to a stoplight and engaged a young boy who first asked if he could wash the windshield. When that was rebuffed by my dad, he simply asked for money. My father gave him a dollar.

Something led my dad to interact with him further. As my father established trust, the young boy told my dad about his situation.

This young man came from a challenging background. He lived in the poorest of slums called 'La Chacarita' in Asuncion, the capital city of Paraguay. The Chacarita was a drug-infested and impoverished area of town known for its gang activity, where literally thousands of people lived in cardboard boxes. He didn't know who his dad was. And like many his age in that area, he belonged to a gang.

That could be the end of the story, but it isn't! After that initial meeting on the street corner in Asuncion, my father began helping this young man out regularly. My father had taken him under his wing—no doubt identifying with his challenging situation—and had become a dad to him.

And when Carlos was in trouble, he would reach out to the man who had shown him love, the man who knew he could become so much more than what his surroundings dictated.

Not long ago, through the tools of social media, I reconnected with Carlos. No, he isn't still trying to wash people's windshields with a greasy rag.

He now lives in Ciudad del Este, Paraguay. He is married, has a family of his own and is pastoring a church, and has a vibrant outreach to the local prison.

Wow, look at the impact that $1.00 and a little time had. Not only in the life of Carlos but now in the lives of countless others.

It affected destiny!

Let's affect destiny together!

Let's give!

"I give best when I give from that deeper place; when I give simply, freely, and generously, and sometimes for no particular reason. I give best when I give from my heart."

Steve Goodier

Chapter 3

Love Elixir

This just happened.

As I am sitting in a local coffee shop working on this chapter, a friend texted me and asked if I was currently in Phoenix. I explained that I was elsewhere working on a fundraising project. He asked how it was going, and I explained that it was proving to be quite a challenging proposition. I went on to tell him more.

The client needed to raise $10m. Generally, at this point in the campaign, we would have already reached about $6m. However, because of some things we discovered after launching, the response to our requests for money was going very slowly. How slowly? Instead of being at $6m, we were only at $650k!

What made this especially challenging was that I had agreed to terms that were not my norm because I really wanted these people to succeed. However, as a result of the snags we had hit, my finances were going to take a massive hit unless I could salvage something from our efforts.

As I expressed this to him, his response was, "Oh, man! That sounds like a challenge, indeed. I am sorry you are going through it. If you need to blow off some steam or just yell at someone – give me a call!"

Wow, his words made me feel so much better.

Did he give me money? No, but he gave me something else I needed. He gave me support, and in so doing, he communicated that he cared. Knowing that he cared lifted my spirits and energized my efforts. All because he gave of his time to reach out to me, ask me how I was, and reminded me that he was there for me.

When you give of your time, ability, or resources to someone in need, you communicate care. Sometimes you may provide indirectly. Sometimes you aren't even giving to what is their 'real need.' But the fact that you are giving expresses care. This is so crucial. We all need to feel cared for, appreciated, and needed.

Sometimes when we have a need, just knowing that someone cares helps us get through – even if they really can't do anything directly about our need.

So a huge benefit of giving is it demonstrates that you care.

If that is true, how do we show that we care?

First, see if you can meet or be a part of meeting the need. If you gave some of your money, time, or ability, could you meet the demand or at least be a part of the solution? That communicates care.

Second, do something unexpected. Most people love a surprise, especially when that surprise is something that helps them or makes their life a little bit easier, if just for a minute. It could be as simple as a card to show appreciation "just because," or offering to watch the kids one night when it wasn't your turn. It could be saying, "Hey, I'll cook dinner tonight" or "Hey, I'll take out the trash," and then just doing it.

Even simple actions can speak volumes, more so if the other person has had an especially difficult day. Imagine if it were your night to cook, but you've had an exceptionally trying and stressful day. Your significant other knows this and offers to cook instead. It's a fantastic expression of caring, even when it may seem too obvious or simple.

Third, sharing is caring. The story is told of an elderly lady who knew her next-door neighbors were experiencing incredibly difficult times. She was at a loss to understand how to help. Their problems seemed so huge and her resources so meager. They needed financial help – she didn't have money. They needed relationship help – she was not a counselor. They needed medical assistance – she was not a doctor. She asked her Pastor for advice. He said, "Bake them a cherry pie each week until they ask you 'Why?'"

She did just that. Baking is one thing she could do. From her meager resources, she scraped together some flour, an egg, and the other ingredients for a crust. She picked cherries from the cherry tree in her back yard, and for the next 9 weeks, she baked pies for her neighbors.

Each week she would take the pie straight from the oven and take it to them. At first, her offering was received hesitantly. After a few weeks, her offering was received suspiciously. By the ninth week, their curiosity was killing them. As the elderly woman rang their bell, they threw open the door and asked,

"Why!? Why are you doing this? Why are you baking us a cherry pie each week?"

The sweet elderly woman responded., "I knew that you
were going through challenging times. And I knew that my resources and abilities couldn't solve your problems. So, I set about showing I cared by baking you cherry pies!"

The couple broke down and cried. They invited the elderly woman in and over a piece of pie expressed how much it meant to them that she was willing to show she cared.

What a powerful opportunity - giving just to show that we care.

Let's give!

"Giving frees us from the familiar territory of our own needs by opening our mind to the unexplained worlds occupied by the needs of others."

Barbara Bush

Chapter 4

Connection is Made

Unfortunately, in our hustle, bustle, get up and get ready, rush the kids out the door, stare at a screen, pull into the garage, pay the bills, microwave a dinner, fall into bed, repeat the next day lifestyles, we miss out on this crucial benefit of the human experience:

Connection

In the novel, 'The Martian', Watney is left stranded and utterly alone on Mars because of several unfortunate oversights and circumstances. While the work of surviving initially keeps him occupied, his days and nights soon become repetitive, boring, and empty. Though Watney rarely says so, many of his actions reveal his desire for human connection. And we don't realize how important that human connection is until we don't have it any longer.

Einstein discovered that two particles that used to be next to each other and were later separated by a significant distance still appeared to maintain a strange kind of connection. Einstein called it "spooky action at a distance."

Quantum physics has now shown that there is a " kind of quantum linkage between all particles, even between those who haven't interacted previously. In fact, they have no idea that the other particle even existed," says Jeff Tollaksen, Director of the Institute for Quantum Studies at Chapman University.

What does that mean to you and me?

It shows that even at our most basic human existence, the smallest particle of who we are is cosmically connected to the other particles of the universe. And when that connection is broken, or strained, or starved, those particles react and yearn for reconnection.

The dangers of isolation are well documented. Studies show that people who feel loved and cared for are actually healthier emotionally, mentally, physically, and spiritually. Allow me to quickly share three studies that have proven this.

Researchers were studying the effect of a diet high in fat and cholesterol in rabbits. One subgroup of rabbits had 60% less atherosclerosis than the group as a whole. Even though they at the same diet. Atherosclerosis, by the way, is the hardening of the arteries and is the leading cause of heart attacks, stroke, and peripheral vascular disease.

They wanted to understand why.

The only notable difference in treatment was one thing. The healthier subgroup was fed and cared for by a lab assistant who took them out of their cages, petted them and talked to them before feeding. (Nerem, Levesque & Cornhill, Science 1980.)

Here are the results of another study done by Medalie and Goldbourt. 10,000 Israeli men were studied and found that those who perceived their wives to be loving and supportive had half the rate of angina of those who felt unloved and unsupported.

Let me finish with this one. A study was done by researchers Russek and Schwartz. They randomly selected 126 healthy young men from Harvard classes and given questions about their perceptions of the love they felt from their parents. Thirty-five years later, 91% of participants who did not perceive themselves to have had a warm relationship with their mothers had diagnosed midlife diseases like coronary artery disease, high blood pressure, duodenal ulcers & alcoholism.

Did you get the connection between all of those studies and their results?

Allow me to take the time to point it out:

In each study, a connection had been created.

And as a result – through that connection - their health was impacted positively. The direct result of a loving connection is an improvement in the well-being of the other person.

Think of that the next time you have the opportunity to connect with someone and show that you care. Not only are you meeting a need. You are impacting destiny, showing care, and making a connection that will improve the health of the person to whom you are generous.

Let's give!

"Generosity is giving good things to others freely and abundantly. Generous behaviors are intended to enhance the well-being of others."

Patricia Snell Herzog

Chapter 5

Doctor Doug

Have you ever wanted to be a doctor? I did! When I was growing up, I was the 'go-to' guy in our family when there was an injury. I can't tell you why this role fell to me, but I remember doctoring stubbed toes, banged shins, and more.

As a young boy, my mother somehow banged her shin pretty badly. I really can't remember how or any specifics about the incident. All I can say is that it took a big gouge of flesh out of her leg. The danger was that the skin on top would heal before the injury deep down by the bone.

Each evening I would care for that wound. After soaking the wound, I would pull back and cut the 'proud flesh' (the skin that was wanting to grow over the injury). Then I would cleanse it with hydrogen peroxide and dress it lightly so that impurities couldn't get in, but some air could.

Another time my mother stubbed her toe pretty severely on a crumbling piece of concrete in our back yard. For some reason, I was given – or took upon myself – the role of taking tweezers and pulling pieces of concrete out of the wound, cleansing it, and bandaging it.

I'm not sure if by telling these stories, I am showing how accident-prone my mother was or how I was the family doctor! And I really don't know why I was the one who took care of these injuries.

But, I think what motivated me most was the desire to help others feel better. In fact, at one point in my life, I considered becoming a Psychologist, and even later, I actually became a Pastor (little known secret about me!). Each of these was motivated by an innate desire to help others know they were loved and cared for.

Well, I never became a Medical Doctor or a Psychologist, and I am no longer a Pastor. But I still am motivated to help others feel loved and cared for. In fact, every night in my journal, I attempt to record one thing, one act that I did for someone else that day to show them that they matter and that I care. I also record one word of affirmation that I said to someone for the same reason.

What I recently discovered was that those acts actually have an impact. To be honest, I was recording them for my own personal measurement to make sure that I was daily giving to others – Acts and Words.

Little did I know that when I gave of my efforts or words to another, I actually was helping them become healthy.

Studies show that those who feel loved and cared for - in other words – when they receive the gift of love from someone else are actually helped emotionally, mentally, physically, and spiritually.

55

Do you remember the three studies that we talked about in the last chapter about the value of connection? Let's look at then again, but from a different angle.

In the first study, researchers were studying the effect of a diet high in fat and cholesterol in rabbits. One subgroup of rabbits had 60% less atherosclerosis (the process which deposits fatty substances, cholesterol, cellular waste products, calcium, and other materials build up in the inner lining of an artery) than the group as a whole – even though they ate the same diet.

The only notable difference in treatment was that the healthier subgroup was fed and cared for by a lab assistant who took them out of their cages, petted them, and talked to them before feeding. (Nerem, Levesque & Cornhill, Science 1980).

Are you serious? If we give someone we care, the indicators which lead to heart attacks are lessened?
Apparently!

56

But wait; there is more proof that we aid in the health of others by giving!

Here are the results of the second study done by Mealie and Goldbourt called "The Israeli Ischemic Heart Disease Study". 10,000 Israeli men were studied and found that those who perceived their wives to be loving and supportive had half the rate of angina of those who felt unloved and unsupported.

And the third one:

Researchers Linda Russek and Gary Schwartz did a study, which they presented by the American Psychosomatic Society. They randomly selected 126 healthy young men from Harvard classes and given questions about their perceptions of the love they felt from their parents. Thirty-five years later, 91% of participants who did not perceive themselves to have had a warm relationship with their mother had diagnosed midlife diseases like coronary artery disease, high blood pressure, duodenal ulcers & alcoholism.

That is powerful!

Did you get the relationship between all of those studies and their results?

Allow me to take this space to point it out:

The rabbits were given affection from their lab attendant.
The 10,000 Israeli men were given love and support from their wives.
The male Harvard students were given love from their parents.

What is the one action that is common in each study?

'Giving'

The rabbits were *given* affection.
The Israeli men were *given* love.
The Harvard students were *given* love.

As a result, their existence was impacted positively.

So whether you want to be a Doctor or not, you and I can still help people be healthier by giving.

Give of your time, abilities, and resources. You choose.

Just give!

"Your Greatness is not what you have, but what you give."

Unknown

Chapter 6

Stress Reliever

I just got off the phone with someone I really care about. Someone who I want to succeed and who I want to help any way that I able. It was a very challenging conversation.

It has been quite a week.

Let me see if I can describe it for you:

I am currently stationed in Washington, D.C., helping a client raise money for a project. To be honest, it isn't going well. We haven't even reached one-tenth of our goal, and we should be at 60%. As you can expect, as a result, stress is high as we try not to point fingers and somehow get our efforts back and figure out how we can make headway.

Along with that, I just got through visiting with my son. I had carved out four days for Thanksgiving and had hoped to spend meaningful, significant time with him in his hometown. Apparently, I did not communicate that well enough and ended up only getting to spend an hour with him. The kicker was that at the end of our hour together, he expressed that he was frustrated because I was never available.

This same week a friend from high school passed away. We had reconnected via social media about a year ago. She told me then that she was dying – and quite honestly, I didn't believe her. For a year, I watched her posts describing her conditions. But because of my past experience with her, I thought she was lying about the whole thing. On Monday, she died. I was overcome with guilt at how I had judged her.

During this same time, a significant project that I have been developing for four years has reached a crucial point in its development. The nitty-gritty of what needs to come together is using more time, energy, and resources than I had budgeted. We may have to push the rollout back – again!

Then the toilet in the apartment broke and totally messed up my already tight schedule - and my apartment floor.

I have also committed to spend an hour each day working on the manuscript for this book. The last thing I have is an hour to give to it. But I must, or I will not meet the completion deadline.

All this capped off with this phone call from my friend. I am committed to investing in this person who lives 3,000 miles away. He really needs my support right now. I am thankful for all the electronic tools to facilitate communication – phone, text, email, Facetime, Skype, Zoom. But none of them can replace face to face dialogue.

Please allow me to add one more very personal component to this scenario:

I hate strained relationships!

But then, who does?

Unfortunately, I feel that I was managing more than my share of relationships that needed special attention. All at the exact same time.

- My work relationships were strained – I needed to take ownership of my part of that.

- My relationship with my son was strained, how could I have communicated better?

- I had unfairly, and incorrectly judged a friend – and now she was dead. Not a lot I can do about that – except forgive myself and try to not be so judgmental next time.

- My publisher was not happy because I was not getting my manuscript written.

- My team was being held back and losing confidence in my leadership because I was not getting my part of our current project developed.

- And now, to top it off, I felt I did not have the time or emotional bandwidth for this close friend right when he needed a little extra!

I've been monitoring my blood pressure, my last reading yesterday was 155/90. Those are definitely not ideal numbers. My head has been pounding from blood being pushed to my brain, apparently in response to the stress. I wonder what my blood pressure is right now.

Back to the phone call that I just finished.

I will confess when I first saw my friend's name on caller ID; my first thought was, "I don't have time for this." I pictured a big black hole that would further be a drain on my energy, emotions, and time. But because I had committed to work through his current issue. I got up from my desk, walked outside (where it is currently 2 degrees wind chill) so that I could have a private conversation. I determined to give the time, energy, and emotions necessary to help him.

What does this have to do with giving?

I did not want to have that conversation. I was stressed to my eyeballs. But I *gave* of my attention, my time, my effort to work through the situation and come out the other side.

I hoped that through the time conversing on the phone, I could *give* my friend the comfort of knowing everything was going to be okay.

When I was done, my friend was comforted, and – even though it took time that I felt I didn't have – my stress was relieved. Yep, in spite of *giving* t what I didn't think I had - I actually relieved *my stress!*

And that is the point of my telling you all of this:

Generosity minimizes stress.

Social psychologist Liz Dunn conducted an experiment. Each participant was given ten dollars. Then they were told they could keep all the money for themselves, or give away as much of it as they wanted.

Dunn found that the more money people gave away, the happier they felt. And, conversely, the more money people kept for themselves, the more shame they experienced.

So, would you like a little less stress in your life?

Then be generous. It can be money, it can be time, it can be ability!

Just give!

"This is the life-giving power of generosity –
doing good to others, simply because you can."

Jan Grace

Chapter 7

Attitude Adjustment

Have you ever had the Blues?

I have, I am certain you have also.

From time to time, I slip into this 'woe is me' attitude that impacts my entire outlook. Most of us have had those times. There was a period in my life I was so overcome with depression that it affected not just my perspective, but also my behavior. I wrote about this in my book 'Overcoming Your Perfect Storm!'.

Depression is not a fun thing.

There are a variety of reasons that someone might suffer from depression. I won't pretend to be a doctor – I don't even play one on television! But I would like to share with you how I dealt with my depression then and what I do now whenever I begin to 'feel blue.'

First, I take a moment to allow myself to admit that I am feeling blue. I used to try to ignore it, hide it, and even deny it. You know the 'fake it till you make it' rule of life. But when I did that, I was only living in denial. So, with the help of a great counselor, I learned that the first step is to admit when I am feeling down.

Second, I try to see if I can identify what is causing me to feel blue. There can be, among other things: physical causes, psychological causes, and moral causes. If there is something I can address that is weighing me down, I do my best to resolve it.

For me, the leading cause for my blueness was and continues to be, that I fixate on things I haven't done, can't do, don't have & can't be. Have you ever done that? One day during my Perfect Storm, I was sitting with a tablet of paper on my lap, pen in my hand, and I was having a hard time coming up with things to be thankful for.

Seriously?

I was having a hard time finding things to be thankful for?

Get this. I was sitting with a tablet of paper on my lap and a pen in my hand. That means I am probably able to read and write. It also means that I had a chair to sit on. It means I was alive! Isn't that enough?

Allow me to paint the whole picture for you.

I was sitting on a balcony on the seventh-floor balcony where I was staying for the next four months. There was a fresh summer breeze blowing across my face, the sun was kissing my cheek. Birds were chirping delightfully just feet from me.

There was a spectacular view to the east where every morning I get to see the sunrise over the mountains. In fact, the whole east wall of my residence was floor-to-ceiling glass. And luscious green plants framed the entire picture.

I had just woken up from a great night's sleep where I didn't have to worry about my safety (unlike my previous place). Nor had I awakened by the resident above me using the restroom at 2 a.m. (also unlike my earlier residence).

I had enjoyed a great smoothie made from fresh fruit and vegetables. I was about to take a warm shower and make myself a delicious cup of coffee.

And yet I was having a hard time finding something to be grateful for.

How can that be?

Here's how:

Somehow I have begun to expect these things. Instead, I was fixating, focusing, meditating on, yearning for, longing for, wishing for all those things I couldn't do, didn't have...... yada, yada, yada.

Which brings us to the third step in how I dealt with my depression. When I recognize that is the cause of my blueness, I identify those things I have to be thankful for. In fact, each evening before retiring for the day, I make a point of writing down three things in my journal for which I can be thankful.

When I stop and identify the many blessings in my life, my perspective changes. And with the adjustment comes a better attitude.

Which brings us to the fourth step in combating the blues and is actually the point of this chapter. Each day I try to do an 'Act of Generosity.' What I mean by that is, each day, I try to either give of my time, ability, or resources to someone who has a need.

It may be a simple act like helping an elderly lady who can't reach something on the top shelf of the grocery store. Or it could be something as big as raising a million dollars for an organization so that it can fulfill its purpose.

It is incredible how my mental health is improved by giving in these ways. Again, each evening, I take a moment and record that Act.

Recently I stumbled across the results of a study that supports this.

The Center for Learning and Occupational Change examined the act of giving by widows to see if their giving yielded beneficial results. Results of that study found that widows who were generous, whether with their time, money, acts, or words, were less likely to have their grief develop into depression. Instead, widows who increased their giving had lower levels of depression in general.

This same study found the same results among dialysis patients. When a dialysis patient practiced generosity, he or she had lower levels of depressive symptoms over time.

Isn't that incredible?

Want to adjust your attitude?

Just give!

"True generosity is an offering, given freely and out of pure love. No strings attached. No expectations."

Suze Orman

Chapter 8

An Apple a Day!

Do you remember that saying, 'An apple a day will keep the doctor away!'? The idea was that if you had an apple a day – yes, a single solitary apple – you would be healthy and never need to see a doctor.

We know apples are indeed good for us. But, I think the Apple Grower's Association came up with that line so they could sell more Granny Smith and Red Delicious.

However, indeed, the main thing you can do to be healthy and live longer is to eat healthy. I like to think that I eat healthy. Although I must admit, I love bacon, and crackers and cheese, and Baked potatoes with tons of butter and sour cream and Nachos with lots of beans and cheese. But other than that, and a few potato chips – I do a pretty good job of eating healthy.

I also love to exercise. Yup, I'm one of the weird ones. I actually like to sweat and strain and feel the burn. I exercise regularly. In fact, one of the first things I do when I travel to a new city to serve a client is to locate the nearest gym.

Now, don't get me wrong – I'm definitely not a 'gym rat,' and I long ago gave up trying to locate my six-pack. I just like to exercise.

They say that exercising is the second main thing you can do to improve your health and live longer. That, for me, is just a nice by-product of working out. I want to believe that I would stay active even if I didn't know that it would benefit my health.

Can I let you in on a little known secret?

There is something else you can do to be healthy and to live longer. Giving of yourself, whether it is time, money, or energy, actually improves your physical health.

Yep, you heard it here first: When you give you actually improve your health, and you will live longer.

Social scientist Stephanie Brown studied a group of older couples for five years and examined the psychological issues surrounding caring and community.

In all, the study examined over four hundred couples. What researchers found was that those couples who provided tangible forms of help to friends, relatives, and neighbors reduced their risk of dying by about one half. This, compared with couples who did not help anyone.

Isn't that incredible? Who would have thought? I mean, eating healthy and exercise seem like no-brainers. Obviously, if you take care of your physical body, it will take care of you.

But giving?

If I give, I am healthier and can expect to live longer? Do you remember the study by Liz Dunn that we talked about in Chapter 6?

Let's review: Social psychologist Liz Dunn conducted an experiment where people were given ten dollars. The recipients were told they could keep all the money for themselves, or they could give away as much of it as they wanted.

Dunn found that the more money people gave away, the happier they felt. And, conversely, the more money people kept for themselves, the more shame they experienced.

The experiment further discovered that the more shame people felt, the higher their cortisol levels rose. Cortisol is generally understood to increase when a person experiences stress. While some cortisol is good, elevated levels of cortisol leads to increased blood sugar – which can lead to diabetes. It can also lead to weight gain and obesity.

Is that crazy or what? There is something inside of me that says 'Give.' When **I don't** give, there is something inside of me that triggers and says, 'Shame on you!'. As a result, my cortisol levels rise, paving the way for weight gain and obesity.

Since that is true, the opposite looks like this:

There is something inside of me that says 'Give. When *I do* give, something inside says, 'Good job!'. My cortisol levels stay down, and I gain a six-pack. Okay, maybe no six-pack – but it is proven that I will definitely be healthier.

So, do you want to be healthy and live to a ripe old age? Maybe we could sit in rocking chairs on the patio and share the stories of the many different ways we gave!

Let's do it.

Let's give!

"Generosity is the most natural outward
expression of an inner attitude of compassion."

Unknown

Chapter 9

Warm Fuzzies

Christmas is my favorite Holiday!

I love it.

Growing up, I would lay on the floor. Put a pillow under my head. Shove my feet under the Christmas tree, and lose myself in the beautiful lights, ornaments, ribbons, and green boughs. I must confess, to this day, I still do this!

Ebenezer Scrooge sure didn't have the same feeling about Christmas.

Do you remember the story written by Charles Dickens? Ebenezer was going through life being mean-spirited and miserly. He refused to give even a pittance to those in need. Responding with "Bah, humbug!" to every wish of a Merry Christmas!

But then, everything changed with the visitation of Ebenezer's dead partner. The ghost declared that, because of Ebenezer's greedy and self-serving life, his spirit was condemned to wander the earth weighed down with heavy chains.

As the story goes, the ghosts of Christmas past, present, and future visited Ebenezer. With each visit, he saw life from a different perspective. He began to understand that his critical outlook and selfishness were robbing him of life itself.

He awoke and changed his life, spending the rest of his days experiencing the euphoria of generosity.

How many times have you been told to do something because 'it is just the right thing to do'? I've great news for you. Being generous is one of those actions that not only is it the right thing to do – it actually gives you the warm fuzzies!

Remember how you felt when someone was generous to you? Maybe they gave you a thoughtful gift. Perhaps they surprised you by mailing you a card. Maybe they babysat for you. Perhaps they took you to a special dinner or a simple coffee.

We have all experienced that warm, fuzzy feeling when we receive goodwill from another person. Did you know that the warm, fuzzy feeling is actually a result of something physiological happening inside of you?

It's the release of something called oxytocin.

Oxytocin is a hormone. It is the hormone that is secreted by a mother during childbirth and nursing. It is sometimes called the "love hormone" because it is also secreted in large doses by a couple during the first six months of their relationship.

Interestingly, it has been discovered that oxytocin is also created when a person receives something special from someone else. That feeling of appreciation you feel is actually a physiological response; it is oxytocin being produced in the body.

And did you know that you can get that same warm, fuzzy feeling when you *give*?

When you are generous, oxytocin is released in your system. The result? The warm fuzzies! And in fact, when you give you actually benefit more physiologically, emotionally, and spiritually than the person who receives your gift.

Her name is Maria.

I didn't know that at first. But there is a lot I didn't realize at first. I just knew that she was in need. Maria cleans the apartments in the building where I was living while on assignment in Chicago.

As I've already told you, my job sends me to various cities where I set up 'house' while I fulfill my assignment. While moving place to place has its difficulties, one of the highlights for me is the opportunity to get to know new people and make new friends.

It is always my intention to learn about my neighbors and allow them to speak into my life as I make myself available to them. Maria was on that list. She was the cleaning lady for the apartment building where I lived.

Each morning I would greet her as I left my apartment on my way to the office. Each evening as I returned, I would stop and ask how her day as she was wrapping up her work.

She would always answer, 'Todo bien!" (It's all good). From the warm, heartfelt smile on her face, I had no reason to not believe her.

One day as I was leaving, I greeted her and received the usual 'It's all good!" As I walked to my car, I noticed her car was only partway into her typical parking space. Half of it was blocking the lane of traffic. As I looked closer, I saw that the front right side of her car was basically sitting on the wheel. The suspension had collapsed.

Something moved inside, and I knew I needed to help. I located her boss and asked him to tell me as much of her story as he could. He was very discrete – but I learned that she was a single mom who had worked for him for over a decade. She was well past what we would consider retirement age.

Among other hardships, her son had recently developed some health issues, and the medical bills were beginning to pile up. She had asked the landlord for as many hours as he could give her. 60 hours a week was his limit. She then picked up another job and worked another 40 there.

As I considered her hardship, I couldn't help but be amazed by her daily sunny disposition and her daily heartfelt 'It's all good!' in response to my morning greeting.

The moment caused me to take personal inventory. What would my response be? Could I say 'It's all good!'? Yes, I have my own set of difficulties – but they seemed to pale in comparison to hers.

I asked him about her car. He said that he had called a tow truck, but that Maria didn't want to lose any work hours, so she was hard at work. He said that he knew for a fact that she did not have money for the repairs.

Although I couldn't take on her medical bills – I did feel like I could take on her auto repair bill so that she could at least get to her jobs and do her best to meet her obligations.

I located the mechanic where the car was towed to and explained the situation that the car's owner was in. I pleaded with him. If at all possible, this car needed to moved to the front of the line. He obliged, and by the end of the day, the car was parked back in its usual spot.

The next morning as I passed her in the hall. I greeted her with a 'Como esta todo?' (How is everything?).

"Todo bien!" she responded with an even warmer heartfelt smile.

Yes, it is all good. Talk about warm fuzzies!

That is why I call Generosity the perfect drug!

That is what Ebenezer Scrooge experienced, and we can experience it too! If you are like me, you can use all the warm fuzzies that you can get in life.

And, here's a bonus, we even produce oxytocin when we simply HEAR about someone giving someone to someone else. Do you feel it? As you read my story, you too got the warm fuzzies!

Maybe that is why the Bible says, "It is more blessed to give than to receive."

So you see it is obvious.

Generosity is the best drug!

Let's give!

"There is no single dollar amount, no particular activity or cause that is better than another, no income level or demographic that matters to generosity, no set variable that is best for giving one's self to another in time of need."

Kathy LeMay

Chapter 10

Chicken or the Egg

According to researcher and author Dan Buettner, the two most vulnerable times in a person's life are the first twelve months after birth and the year following retirement.

You have probably heard stories about perfectly healthy individuals who died shortly after they retired from a lifelong career.

Some researchers suspect that for these people, the end of their career also signified the end of their purpose in life, which affected their health and well-being.

A study or retired employees of Shell Oil found that men and women who retired early (age 55) were more likely to die earlier than those who retired at age 65.

A similar study of almost 17,000 healthy Greeks showed that the risk of death increased by 51% after retirement. These two studies suggest that there may be some risk involved when defining self by one's career.

It seems crucial to reshape life's big questions and find ways to continue serving a purpose, even after retirement, to improve the chances of a longer, healthier life.

However, retirement is not the only time that we question our purpose. Quite honestly, it can haunt us at any stage of our lives.

When we are in grade school and have more questions than answers, and everyone is larger than us and telling us what to do: We might ask, "What is my purpose?"

During High school, when we don't fit in, and we can't impress, and we don't measure up: We might ask, "What is my purpose?"

As we graduate from College and can't land a job that matches what we have a diploma in: We might ask, "What is my purpose?"

As we face the day-to-day stresses of caring for and raising toddlers who can't reason with us and seem to only make messes and fuss: We might ask, "What is my purpose?"

When we get up at 0 dark thirty every day, make our way to work, sit in our cubicle day after day for years: We might ask, "What is my purpose?"

When we lay in our bed at hospice, trying hard to pull in one more breath: We might ask, "What was my purpose?"

Without purpose, we lose life. Lack of purpose is actually the leading cause of boredom, addiction, depression, aggression, and even suicide. Unfortunately, many misplace 'purpose' with 'pleasure', which quite honestly is just 'escapism.'

Surprisingly, if we seek purpose through pleasure, we actually have poorer health. Studies show that people who find joy only in pleasing themselves have higher incidents of inflammation and are more susceptible to viruses and antibodies.

"Doing good and feeling good have very different effects on the human genome, even though they generate similar levels of positive emotion," says study researcher Steven Cole, professor of medicine at the University of California, Los Angeles, and a member of the University's Cousins Center for Psychoneuroimmunology.

He continued, "Apparently, the human genome is much more sensitive to different ways of achieving happiness than our conscious minds."

Could this be another reason why the Bible tells us, "It is better to give than to receive?"

Doing something meaningful and helpful brings emotional and psychological benefits to your life. It brings health, it brings life, it gets you up in the morning!

Somehow, when we are generous, we start believing in ourselves. It somehow seems to justify our existence. We begin to realize that we are needed! We say to ourselves, "Without me, this wouldn't happen!"

Science has confirmed the healthy benefit of having purpose. Having a strong sense of purpose can also help you:

Live longer. In a study of over 73,000 Japanese men and women, Dan Buettner (Blue Zones) found that those who had a secure connection to their sense of purpose tended to live longer than those who didn't. Additionally, he identified the factors that most centenarians share, _one of them being a strong sense of purpose._

Protect against heart disease. Another study in 2008 found that a lower level of purpose in Japanese men was associated wit earlier death and cardiovascular disease. More research in this areashowed that "purpose is a possible protective factor against near future myocardial infraction among those with coronary heart disease."

Prevent Alzheimer's disease. In studies of thousands of elderly subjects, Dr. Patricia Boyle, a neuropsychologist at the Rush Alzheimer's Disease Center in Chicago found that people with a low sense of life purpose were 2.4 times more likely to get Alzheimer's Disease than those with a strong purpose. Further, people with purpose were less likely to develop impairments in daily living and mobility disabilities.

Handle pain better. Purpose can also positively affect pain management—a study in *The Journal of Pain* found that women with a stronger sense of purpose were better able to withstand heat and cold stimuli applied to their skin.

Have better relationships. In 2009, Richard Leider teamed up with Met Life to assess the purpose of over 1,000 adults. They found that those with a high sense of meaning in their lives spent more time and attention on their loved ones and communities On the whole, people with purpose tend to be more engaged with their families, colleagues, and neighbors, enjoying more satisfying relationships as a result.

All of this reminds me of the age-old question. Which came first the Chicken or the Egg? If it was the egg, where did the egg come from, and who kept the egg warm so that it would hatch? If it was the chicken, where did it come from? Did it appear as an adult, or was it a chick first?

The same could be said about purpose and generosity.

Which comes first, finding that giving is your purpose or giving so that you have purpose?

The answer is "yes"!

Just give!

"To be a generous person, you must act. Generosity is a practice. And as with anything we practice, we get better at it over time."

Barbara Bonner

Bonus Chapter

5 Generosity Stories for your Benefit

RAKs

From my friend Kim Cox-Simister

Recently, my husband and I celebrated our Sixth Year Anniversary with our friends.

Really not having any idea what we could do, I stumbled across something from Pinterest. It was a Service Scavenger Hunt.

Basically, it consisted of giving our friends a list of Random Acts of Kindness, and whoever finished the list the fastest, won.

Actually, everyone who did anything on the list won, because they are just awesome like that!

We had three teams; six adults and five children, between the ages of seventeen and eleven.

They started at 12:30, and they had until 4:00 to complete it. They were encouraged to post lots of pictures to our event page so everyone could could follow along on their journeys.

The stories we heard, were awesome and interesting.

From all three teams, we heard the most challenging was helping someone take their groceries to their car. I have to admit, I thought that one might be.

People just don't trust people anymore. They wonder what the alternative motive is. But even when it was explained they where performing Random Acts of Kindness, they were still turned down.

We don't need your kindness here...how sad.

One team got super creative and instead of "playing a board game with someone in a nursing home", they found some seniors hanging outside their homes and did magic tricks for them.

It made their day!

Before they left, they also helped pull some weeds and picked up trash.

Reading some of the posts and seeing their pictures, would cause me to tear up.

One of the pictures was of my daughter leaving a sticky note on a public restroom mirror that said, "You're beautiful".

You sure are!

Some of the teams took my list as more of a suggestion, and went totally rogue on their own.

That was awesome.

One of which was a couple, who after meeting a cashier from the day before at a big box store, found out she was a struggling mom who was recently diagnosed with a life threatening health condition, went back to track her down to give her a gift of encouragement.

She wasn't at her place of employment this day, but I think it kind of worked out for the best, anyway.

While asking for the employee, it was brought to the teams attention that even if she was there, under no circumstances would she be allowed to accept any gifts.

Doing so would warrant immediate termination.

Bound to not give up, the team sought out the acting manager to try to sweet talk an exception.

I am proud to say, THEY WERE SUCCESSFUL!

Wow! Random Acts of Kindness sounds so simple, and yet sometimes is not easy.

Who would have thought?

I can't say who was more inspired by the activities, the recipients or the teams. Many of the RAKs were anonymous. But there are reports of kids who where approached in a store, climbing out of their seat to stick their heads out the car windows to yell, "THANK YOU!", once they recognize the team in the parking lot. I think that's a win.

Upon reaching the finish line, teams were bubbling with smiles and stories to tell.
It was a beautifully, great day!

I was so honored our friends would do this for us.

We didn't want gifts. We didn't want praise. We just wanted others to feel love and to spread it.

I think it was pretty successful.

Would we do it again? Well heck yeah! I've already got another list started.

But this time, I want in on giving!

Simple Kindnesses Can Change The World

From my friend Fulton Breen

In the fall of 1974, I was beginning to realize that I'd have to make a decision about attending college or not, and if so, what college. The challenge of how to get accepted, and even more daunting, how to pay for it, hadn't yet reached consciousness yet. I had taken the SAT during my junior year and if I recall, I barely broke 1,000, 1,100 tops, as my score. I needed to take it again but that takes money so I decided to stick with what I had and let my future alma mater be decided by fate. This seems reckless as I think of it now but there was no one to coach me about this stuff at the time. Also, going to college was not expected of

118

me; it wasn't discouraged by any means, it was simply a choice that was left up to me.

My four sisters and I enjoyed a good childhood. Our modest upbringing encouraged independence while structure was provided through family rules and strict weekly attendance at Mass. My father struggled with alcohol with my mother keeping us afloat working night shifts while attending school to earn her nursing degree. In retrospect, I consider the experiences and lessons learned during this period to be some of the most valuable and rewarding of my formative years. However, at the time, all I recall was the desire to "get away" and college seemed to provide the opportunity to do that.

Most of my friends were going to Georgia Tech, the University of Georgia and Davidson as I recall. Although I had many friends in high school, I remember wanting to start from scratch; go someplace different. Clemson entered my short list of possibilities when I inquired about a football pennant hanging in my cousin's bedroom. He was a Georgia Tech graduate and explained that Clemson was a respected school located in South Carolina. For some reason I locked on to Clemson as my choice from that point on. I had never visited Clemson, didn't know of anyone that had been there and had no idea of what they offered. Apparently, intuition was a powerful influence in my decision process as Clemson's was the only application I sent.

I distinctly recall that there was an $80 application fee, which I borrowed, that in turn brought to the forefront the issue of "how am I going to pay for this if I get in?." The going pay scale was roughly $3.00 an hour so sheer numbers of hours wasn't going to be an easy solution to this problem. I worked three jobs that summer; golf course maintenance, Greenhouse/flower shop and as a janitor.

By mid-August, I had enough saved to pay for tuition, room and a 5-day meal plan; I figured I'd just "wing it" for food on the weekends. As I had no car, I couldn't participate in the orientation programs offered during the summer, I just showed up the weekend before classes began the following Wednesday. I recall packing a box full of all my necessary items and taking Amtrak for $10.75 one way from Atlanta to Clemson. By the end of that first Saturday, I had checked in and began to relish the idea of being in college...

Monday morning brought the realization that I had to register for classes with all the other latecomers. I distinctly recall the flurry of activity to sign up for elective courses that were easy and possibly even fun. Advice about these electives carried all the validity of a stock recommendation on the subway but somehow I ended up with Entomology 101 under Dr. Tom Skelton.

On Wednesday, the first day of class, Ent 101 professor Tom Skelton captured our attention immediately with his confident and enthusiastic personality. In an effort to gauge our understanding of entomology and agriculture in general, Dr. Skelton asked questions of the class throughout his opening statements about the syllabus and expectations for the semester ahead. I recall answering one of the questions that had no other potential respondents: "Who knows what a 'systemic pesticide' is"? Having worked in summer jobs where pesticides were used, I knew the answer and basked in the delivery of my correct response. After class, Dr. Skelton called me over to speak with him. He proceeded to ask me my declared major, "Microbiology" I responded. "Why microbiology?" came his counter. "I don't know", my voice trailing off. As if it were decided already, he concluded "I want you to major in entomology".

A dynamic middle-aged man paying attention to me at this stage in my life, when I needed it most, resulted in an immediate "ok" thereby inaugurating the first step in my new life.

By the end of my first semester, it became clear that my new mentor had much more in mind for me than to just guide me through basic entomology. With Dr. Skelton's connections I was provided the means to pay for my second semester including a 7 day meal plan! In fact, I never paid another nickel for my remaining three years of school.

For reasons I can only begin to understand now as I approach my 59th birthday, this man changed my life forever with his kindness and attentiveness. Dr. Skelton's simple act of charity radically changed the course of my life forever yet he did so with absolutely no possible benefit for himself in mind. My life is full of people doing these sorts of things as I'm sure is yours. Why do people do these beautiful things for others...others they may not even know and the impact they may never see?

I believe that we all are the beneficiaries of these kindnesses. If we think about it, the half-dozen or so pivotal people and events in all of our lives that have led to who we are today may likely have appeared insignificant at the time. The haphazard introduction to a friend of a friend who eventually becomes your spouse, the compliment from a stranger that awakens your desire to develop a latent talent, the smile offered to a stranger that changes their day.

Who can say which of these acts will set the course of another's day and maybe their life?

These kindnesses "cost" you nothing yet often result in a critical milestone in someone's life. Imagine the impact of making a habit of offering simple kindnesses, mentorship or affirmations to those we encounter each day knowing that some percentage, albeit small, will change their life for the good. Aristotle once said, "We are what we repeatedly do. Excellence, then, is not an act, but a habit." Make kindness a habit and know that you are changing the world, even if the change isn't immediately seen.

I want credit!

Submitted by Doug Clark

Would you like a receipt for your donation this morning?

A torn blanket, a broken lamp, a badly damaged chest of drawers were some items in better condition. That is what I discovered one morning as I drove up to my local Goodwill drop-off location piled by the drop-off dock.

I was downsizing. After giving the bulk of my stuff away to friends and selling a few other items to strangers, I was generously donating what remained to Goodwill Industries.

As you are aware, Goodwill Industries helps people with barriers to employment learn skills to find competitive employment. One of the ways they do this is by operating stores where used items that have been donated are sold.

At the risk of being considered a dumpster diver, I started poking through the pile. The items I discovered as I dug deeper were in even worse condition.

My first thought, I must admit was incredibly judgmental. How could people just leave junk here? It was obvious to me that it was stuff that they just couldn't get rid of any other way.....

Oh wait! Wasn't that what I was doing?

I had given my best away to my friends, sold some stuff to strangers, and now I was dumping off the stuff that nobody wanted.
Yes, dumping.

I tried to justify in my mind that I was being incredibly generous. That what I was doing would help someone in their training to find competitive employment. Really? What kind of employment? What kind of skills?

I could see it now on their job application. "Past job experience: I learned how to identify junk and carry it to the dumpster."

Was I really being generous? A simple definition of generosity that I like is:

Generosity: the willingness to give others something of value.

There is an old adage that says: "One Person's junk is another Person's treasure."

126

Yes, I could say I was giving. But I would have to be honest, it was just junk. Yes, using some kind of metric what I was giving could be seen as valuable to someone. And yes, some benefit would result from my donation.

But I had definitely inflated the value of what I was giving to justify my actions.

As the clerk offered me a charitable giving receipt for my donation, I decided then and there to correctly measure what I was doing and minimize the philanthropic weight that I had put on my activity. Symbolically, as a first step toward this, I said, "No, thank you."

Shirt off My Back!
Part 1

Submitted by Doug Clark

I lost my shirt last night....well I didn't actually lose it, I gave it away. Let me explain. While I was in the local big box store last night, I walked by a mom, her daughter and her teen aged son and as I did the son pointed to me and said, "That is a beautiful shirt!"

He obviously had good taste, as it was one of my favorites. A silk, Tommy Bahama style shirt that I had just acquired two weeks before. In fact, it was the first time that I had worn it.

He repeated again, 'Wow, that is a great shirt!" I was struck with the innocence and the honesty with which he made his declaration. Immediately, I was overcome with the desire to give him the shirt.

I turned toward him and asked, "Do you want it?" He looked at me, not knowing how to answer. He kind of stuttered as he admitted, "Y-Y-Y-Yeah, I would love to have that shirt!"

I began unbuttoning my shirt and said, "It's yours!". Incredulously he said, "Really, are you serious?" I said, "Yes, I just ask that you give me your shirt (a basic white t-shirt) so that I can finish my shopping."

He couldn't believe it. Neither could his mom. Nor his sister. Nor could I!

As we exchanged shirts in the dairy section, the young man started repeatedly saying, "Thank you so much, thank you so much, thank you so much! It is so beautiful!" His mother chimed in, "Oh my God, thank you. That is so kind." His sister stood there speechless, mouth wide open, just taking it in.

"You are very welcome." I replied. I could not believe the feelings that were flooding me. It was surreal. Like a natural high. Warm fuzzies is what some would call it. Scientists have identified it as oxytocin: commonly known as the 'love hormone'. It is the hormone that a mother secretes when nursing (and interestingly that a new couple feels during their first six months of courtship). When you give, your body actually secretes that same hormone!

I slipped his t-shirt on and walked away. As I did so I realized that our exchange had drawn a crowd. I made my way through the group that

129

had collected, finished my shopping and went home. For the rest of the evening I marveled at what had just transpired and celebrated the exchange that I had just had the privilege of participating in.

Shirt Off My Back
Part 2

Submitted by Doug Clark

I was standing in the kitchen cooking breakfast. He was standing by the breakfast island waiting to be served.

"Man I love that shirt!" he exclaimed.

"I" am, well, you know who I am.
"He" is a young 18 year old friend - who will remain nameless.

My priority for the last two months has been to speak into the life of this young, big hearted, easily conflicted young man. It has had its moments. There have been times when he has opened up and received words of love, guidance and wisdom. Other Times when he has lashed out in anger, fear and ignorance.

My role has been a drop in the bucket compared to what others have contributed. Among them, his parents have made it their priority to speak into his life for the last 13 plus years. They have modeled true love to him: generosity, consistency, patience, gentleness, firmness, forgiveness, and instruction.

The challenge has been to try and figure out what is going on in his young mind and heart, gain his trust and gently show him a better Way. Each night I compare notes with his parents.

Are we getting anywhere? Are we making progress? Sometimes there are small glimmers of hope. Other times we our hearts are bleeding, having been slashed open by words that he has spoken in a heated moment.

I peel the shirt off my back and handed it to me. He looks at me in awe and appreciation.

These two months have flown by. I am emotionally exhausted. I can't imagine how his parents must feel. Because they have chosen to not make his actions public – few will truly understand what they have gone through.

It is time for me to leave. I must get on with my life. Have I made an impact? Will he see how much he is loved? Will open his heart and trust?

Two days later he leaves. Moves out. Without a thank you to those who have loved him for years. He's 18, he's free to go where he wants, and he does. Will he recognize that he has truly experienced love? I don't know, the story isn't completely written yet.

I do know this. Love is a gift. Love is a challenge. Love is inconvenient. Love can hurt. Love has no guarantees. Love can have no strings attached. Yet, love we must! For truly that is the essence of Life. It is the essence of God. God is Love.

Are you giving the gift of Love today? Please do. Don't quit. The story isn't completely written yet.

Have you identified and appreciated who has Loved you? Please do. They are longing for a happy ending to the story.

AFTERWARD

Well there you have it, the incredible benefits of the perfect drug: Generosity!

Hopefully after reading this book you too want to experience the incredible benefits of living a generous life.

I encourage you to join us.

A generous life is the most exciting way to live. For it is in giving and serving that we truly come alive.

We would love to help you live a passionately generous life. Check out our website: www.GiveServeLive.com.

In it we have projects you can give to, along with various tools and resources to assist you in your desire to be generous.

Made in the USA
Monee, IL
18 April 2022